The Book of Hope

The Book of Hope

Bishop Christopher Wiggins

To order additional copies of this book, contact:
Xlibris Corporation
1-888-795-4274
www.Xlibris.com
Orders@Xlibris.com
85046

CONTENTS

PREFACE

My name is Chris Wiggins, and I was born with Cerebral Palsy but I am thankful for that gift. God has been so good to me. He has been my hope since birth. I have also fought with depression. I have learned that medications are not the only things that help. The other thing that helps is the work of God. When Jesus was took to the wilderness to be tempted by Satin he said "If you are the son of God turn this stone into bread" and Jesus replied "It is written you shall not live on bread alone but by every word that is perceived out of the mouth of God." I would eventually learn that the word is what I would need. I have also begun to understand that God and only God is the true answer. Circumstances in life that happen to you do not necessarily mean you have done anything wrong. I began to understand as you will find from reading this book that situations in life were to build character. People and things sometimes are sent to prepare you for your purpose.

ACKNOWLEDGEMENTS

A special thanks to Ten Lakes Staff you are number one. To Dr. Z. I say Thank you from the bottom of my heart. To Iron Mike you packed a punch in caring and I say thanks. To Sara I also say thank you, you encouraged me to keep writing. To Akron General Medical Center thanks to units 6100 and 6400 for caring a lot for my depression. Thanks to Blick Clinic Dr. Quant you helped me when I was young. You are great, caring and understanding. Your tough love got me thru a lot. Dr Aurora you have never expected anything but the best. Sara McClain working with you I am reminded of what's important and that is my faith in God. In hard times she always tells me to "ask your heart" and when I do I find it easy to reach my soul and spirit man. Another person that has encouraged me in my writing is Tonia Bogema, she has supported me with my writing along with many others from Blick Clinic. Now Support Care friends, starting with my good friend Dee, she is a kind person who encouraged me with my writing. She is the one that first challenged me to dig deep and become the writer I am today. Brandy Pine is like a sister to me; her tough but kind love has taught me to perciver in hard situations. I am also thankful to the rest of the Support Care Family. To Bishop, Apostle Bibie I am very grateful for him and his wife. They are like family. He has shown me true love and for that I am grateful. Now United Disability Services has Liz Price who has taught me to respect myself and not be so quick tempered. Lastly is Middlebury Manor, to the people there thanks a bunch. To Minnie I say thank you, you have taught me the importance of keeping your word. Because now I know that's how people measure a man.

CHAPTER ONE

The Early
Years

I was born to the parents of Charles and Teresa Wiggins. Due to challenges and complications I was born 3 months prematurely. Due to my Cerebral Palsy (CP) and impairment that I mentioned earlier I would sometimes quit breathing as a baby.

After getting the CP under control temporarily for a year I became CP's states poster child. As a poster child I would meet many famous celebrities such as Lou Ferrigno who played the Incredible Hulk. At the age of 2 ½ I would go to foster care. While in foster care I would have severe behavioral problems and would bounce from home to home. But later on in life I figured out that my actions came from a rebellious spirit with in me.

As the bible says "that that is spirit is spirit and that that is flesh is flesh." I didn't vision this in my past years, but I would realize later on in life that I have a significant purpose in life. During my childhood I had hate for the condition that I once believed God had done to me. This way of thinking would put me in a position to where I would have thoughts of suicide.

NOTES

NOTES

CHAPTER TWO

The Search Begins

Being rebellious and having suicidal tendencies where nothing but evil spirits trying to overcome me. During my teen years I would always wonder what my purpose in life was. I would wonder what the lord could ever do with me.

Then once I got to listen to a well known preacher at the time by the name of Rod Parsley. He read a scripture from the word of God that stuck with me forever. "God uses the foolish to confine the wise and the poor to confine the rich." Around this time in my life various people of "faith" would tell me that I have a gift. Those saying this made me more curious into finding out what my gift in life was.

When I turned sixteen I began to realize when dealing with religion you have to be careful who you discuss it with. In this time of searching I started to understand you have to be cautious on what you read, hear, and say! People of faith would tell me to watch what type of people I accompany myself with. I later learned that not praying and having faith can lead to being easily persuaded by people with evil spirits.

Once I turned seventeen my eagerness began to get out of control. To those reading this book I want to tell you that the more you study the word of God, the more Satan will throw obstacles in front of you. But hopefully these scriptures will give you more encouragement in Christ our Savior. In the scriptures of God the Bible reads that "No weapon formed against me will prosper." Another scripture is "I can do all things through Christ that strengthens me!"

NOTES

NOTES

CHAPTER THREE

The Purpose was revealed

At the age of 18, I began to have a severe drug and alcohol problem. It didn't matter to me that it was illegal nor did I think about the consequences I could endure.

One night while out drinking due to a severe alcohol problem my purpose was revealed to me. I would drink after taking my medication. I realized eventullay that night after I came from my hangover what people were talking about. While I was sitting at home the sprit of the lord came to me and said u are to preach the word of god the spirit of the Lord would come to me. Thus, revealing my purpose in life.

The spirit of the Lord said to me "You shall not die, but you shall preach the Gospel around the world." I began realizing a couple days later that I had a job to do but I had still a lot of things to deal wit in my life. I began pondering the thought to myself "how could God use someone like me?" As the Bible says "God will bring things back to your remembrance." I began to remember the scripture that Rod Parsley had said. . "God uses the foolish to confound the wise and the poor to confine the rich." Then I began to think, could I be the foolish to confine the wise?

People looked at me as a man with a challenge sitting in a chair, but not as an upright man. It is important to realize that no matter your mental or physical condition if you believe in God with all your heart you are an upright man or woman of God. It is truly all within the spirit. The Bible says "We are to worship God in spirit and in truth." Too many people think about the physical man but we need to also think of the spiritual man. I would learn this later in life.

NOTES

NOTES

CHAPTER FOUR

Fighting the Enemy Within

After learning my purpose I happen to deal with a substantial number of obstacles in my life. Eventually, I would begin to understand that these obstacles were only spirits trying to pull me down to there level. It is also imperative to understand that some of the things we struggle with we happen to bring upon ourselves.

I figured that a lot of reasons why I was having troubles and the spirits of the enemy were chasing me was because I was not truly into the word of god. I found out that this way of life is an actual "lifestyle", that means we are to live the way Christ lived. It doesn't mean just going to church or reading a glimpse of your bible, when at church it Is important to take NOTES of what the sermon is about. While reading the scriptures of the qbible we need to study it with passion for the word of God. It is also good to ask God for revelations and knowledge for we can understand the word of God. The bible states "study to show self approved a workman is not to be ashamed rather to divide the word of truth. As I began to understand these things it got harder and harder to fight within. Again, the behavior problems started which would delay me of my calling.

I would not know the significants of the holy spirits in my life. I would later on in life learn that know matter how hard you try to pull away from your calling God will make sure you reach your calling in life. No matter if you or I are equipped for the calling, Bishop William Bibbie my fateher would always say "those who God call on he will equip".

I didn't understand that the problems that aroused once again would actually lead to me meet a mighty man of God. These problems such as fornication, lying on my caregivers, and outrageous out burst would try to derail my path into meeting this wonderful man.

NOTES

NOTES

NOTES

NOTES

CHAPTER FIVE

An Angel in the Flesh

Two words come to mind when I describe William Bibbie, teacher and believer. From day one he had faith in me even when I didn't have faith in myself. Meeting him was a blessing in disguise. One of the caregiver in my apartment introduce me to Connie Riley who would later introduce me Bishop William Bibbie.

Not evening knowing me he whispered you will preach the word. From that day forward a lot of times I would preach with a slogan "get your junk out the trunk" because as I began to preach I realized why I didn't understand my calling in the past. There was too much "junk in my trunk".

What God meant for good I was turning it around and making it bad. But William Bibbie and his wife Joanne who I call mom. Told me that the wheelchair is my "platform". I writing this book to let everyone know that there weakness is really there strength.

Because what we think is making us weaker is really making us stronger. Then a few months later and sitting by him and watch how the ministry unfolds, he told me he would ordain me. Eventually I would become the youth pastor of New covenant ministries of America incorporated. After a year went by I started my own church named Breakthrough today Ministries.

NOTES

NOTES

CHAPTER SIX

The Bishop Within

In 2006 i became bishop of breakthrough today ministries and united disabled Christian association. Even though in UDCA is still in works I'm teaching the disabled Christians that there disabilities is not a disability but a challenge from God.

Again I refer to a scripture mentioned earlier "God uses the foolish to confound the wise and the poor to confound the rich". I truly believe with every fiber of my being that my life came out perfect. Perfect, because in Gods time his plan did take place.

It' very important that even though we go through bumps and bruises, we know as long as we follow the blueprint for our lives set by God, we will be successful.

NOTES

NOTES

CHAPTER SEVEN

In memory of my best friend

While I was ministering at university park, I came across a very good friend name Munroe King. His friendship, in my opinion, would be the greatest friendship I would have. I was amazed by him and his ability to preach the word of God. To this day I truly believe that he set the standard in being a best friend and minister, he set the bar high. I can remember when I first started practicing to become a minister, he told me you either do it or don't.

There is something I would love forever about that man and that is that he had a very severe sickness but that would not bring him down. Every time I think about feeling sorry for myself I think about the courage he had possessed that kept him going each day. I ask God to possess me with that same gift as I preach the word of God. In his memory I will encourage others to follow the word God as he did me.

NOTES

NOTES

CHAPTER EIGHT

Poetry from the heart

wheeling in a chair
preaching all day
hoping the enemy
gets out of my way
as a chair as my car
and the bible for fuel
I'm going to make the devil
Look like a fool
Teaching and preach all of the day
Knowing life is a school
More then one way
So as I come to a closure
With this poem you see
I move ahead forward
And keep satan behind me

Blasting off

Blasting off 1.2.3 . . .
Here I come
With good news for thee
The lord is your savior
And word is your launch pad
Oh yes! That's true
God has love for one and all
And has hope that we stand tall
All together for the lord
So his kingdom
Can be on one accord

the lords heart is calling
for one in all
and Jesus arms are open wide
saying come on in
and let me be your guide
my heart is calling for each of you
my heart is calling oh yes it is true
knocking on the doors
to our heart because the lord
wants to give your souls a jump start

Labor for the lord

Laboring for the lord that's
What I'm trying to do
Riding this book of hope
For each one of you
Trying be a Shepard to one in all
Showing even the ones
In wheelchairs can stand tall
His grace and mercy does abide
That's what we should always
Use as our guide

Wheeling for Jesus

Wheeling for Jesus is what I am
Going to do
Wheeling for Jesus through and through
When I see people sad and depress
I tell them that's just the devil's mess
To get them confused and all off track
I give them the word of God to
Keep satan off there back
Wheeling for jesus is what I'm going
To do so that's what I'm going to
Encourage for all of you

The light is on

The light is on
Oh yesiree!
Because I turned to God
You see!
I learned no matter
What I go through
Jesus Christ knows
What to do

The House of God

The house of God
A place to dwell
When it seems like nothing
Is going well
This place is calm
And smell so sweet
The things that happen
Inside are oh so neat
The house of God
A place to dwell
When everything is not
Going well

Battling with Depression

Battling with depression
I am reminded each day
To smell the roses
And to read the word
Of God is the only way
It goes away
Battling with depression
It's not really pain
I look at it as something
I've gained
It teaches me to love
It teaches me to care
Most of all
I know God will be there

Life's lessons

Life lesson is sometimes hard
Life's lesson is sometimes sweet
But its is really neat
Sometimes you have victory
Sometime you have pain
Sometimes you're a loser
And sometimes you'll gain
But through it all God is there
To lead you the right way
So when you wake up in the morning and wake up at night
This is what you say
O,dear God thank you for today
Thank you for what you gave and taken away

Time has come

The time has come
To welcome him in
Jesus Christ our savior
Our partner within!
The time has come to draw so close
To the lord that you get the holy ghost
The time has come to praise his name
All around the land
Because remember
He is the only one who can save
Girl, boy, woman, or man

Singing to the lord

Singing to the lord
With praises abound
Singing with the lord takes the pain away
It's such a gift that the lord does love
It makes the angels smile
From up above
Make a joyful noise! Onto
The lord and that will keep
God's people on one accord

Medecine for the soul
That is the word of the lord
It gets a through each and everyday
It guides us when were out at bay
But medicine of the soul is the word lord
It is the spiritual sword

Your soul is a city and it houses your sprit
To many people don't even dig it
There worried about the flesh on thee
There not worried about the cavery
What happen on the hill that day
To keep the enemy away
The soul is a city so often over looked
And people mines and hearts are getting fried and
cooked because there not pay
Attention to the truth in hand
We have limited time on this land

LIFE IS NOT A GAME
WITH IT WE NEED TO
BE TRUE
AND READ THE
WORD OF THE LORD
FROM GOD SO
WE CAN BE ON
ONE A CORD

THE BREAKFAST OF CHAMPIONS
IS THE WORD OF THE LORD
IF YOU START YOUR DAY
WITH IT YOU AND GOD
WILL BE ON ONE
A CORD

THE GREAT POSITION
IS THE LORD I'M THANKFUL
FOR HIS WORD
WHICH IS A SPRITIUAL
TWO EDGED SWORDS
BY HIS STRIPES I AM HEALED AND
THANKS TO HIS BLOOD MY SINS
ARE SEALED

The mind is your battle ground
you store things in your mind like u
Do a floppy and the devil job
Is to remind u what u did sloppy
The devil will play with u in your mind
Make u think that bad is good and
Good is not fine he will tease u
And make jokes of your life
That's when you need to use the word the 2 edged sword as your knife

The race is given to the swift
The bible is cool and nift
The bible is weights for are soul to lift
To keep in shape and be on track
And beat the devil in the back

Stay in on one accord that is what we need
To do so we can stand with one
Another to make the devil blue
As brothers and sisters and children of god
we need to look past this world and start looking beyond

plouting the air is not the way of god
we need to make it safe the world is ours to
borrow and were only passing through
that's why we need to lean to the word
of god to know what to do
the enviorment is special it is an awesome gift

STUDY THE WORD
TO STAY INTUNE
WITH THE ONE
THAT HUNG
THE MOON
STUDY THE WORD
OF THE LORD
SO EVERYONE
JUMP ON BORD

GOD CARRIES THE LOAD
FOR YOU AND ME
THAT'S WHY HE
GAVE US JESUS
TO SAT THE
CAPTIVES FREE
GOD CARRIES THE LOAD
O YES INDEED

FOR ME AND MY HOUSE
WHE SHALL SERVE
THE LORD
HE IS THE
ONE THAT
KEEPS ME
AND GOD
ON ONE A CORD
I THANK GOD
THAT HE'S
MY SAVIOUR
AND LORD

IT DRIVE'SME TO THE LORD
I'M TALKING ABOUT
THE WORD OF GOD
I HOLD IT NEAR
TO MY HEART
EACH AND EVERY
DAY
I UNDERSTAND
HIS WORD IS
THE TRUE
WAY

IT'S NOT BUINESS AS USUAL
WE ARE AT THE IN TIMES
YOU SEE
THE LORD IS
COMING FOR
YOU AND ME
TO TAKE US
TO ARE PLACE IN GLORY

TIME TO XAMINE OURSELF
THE WOURLD IS COMING
TO AN END
WE NEED TO
KNOW THAT JESUS
IS OUR ONLY
TRUE FRIEND

WE CAN NOT CLIMB A TOWER
TO THE THROWN OF GRACE
WE NEED THE HOLY SPIRIT
TO SEEK HE'S
FACE

The home is not made of a building
It is made of the word of god
To use that as a foundation
For all the world to live up on
The home is not a building it is the thrown of grace cause if god is not in it
With the lord we will not win it
And are mind would be it to space

NOTES

NOTES

CHAPTER NINE

The Blessing's From God In My Life

At the time I became a bishop I started to appear on television.
I have been told that I am unique, because of the fact that
I'm one of the few bishops that has C.P. or a
nether disability since berth. I thank God for that apratoneaty

Another blessing that I thank god for is
I have a better since of revelation and knowledge for the word of
God. Previously in the book I had mentioned Bishop and pastor Bibbie. I
mentioned that they are like family but I am so grateful to say he is the only
closes thing to a father I've had. To my mother I am very thankful to you
and the upbringing you gave to me. In this book I am apologizing from the
bottom or my heart for all the wrong I have done to you. Your only wish
in life was to have respectable children. My goal at this point is to give you
that. To my grandmother on my father side, you were there for me when I
was young, I thank you for that and it is my goal to do better in life then
what I did as a child.

NOTES

NOTES

CHAPTER TEN

How I Met The Love Of My Life

Her name is Millie Zender she has been with me threw thick in thin I thank god for her she is my best friend there are been times in my life where we did not see eye to eye I was with her once before but I did not realize what a good thing I had we met at our work place United Disability Services for along time we were together but I did not treasure the gift that god gave to me and her now we are back together and to her I say u are a special person and I love you very much you showed me a lot about myself and the true meaning of love as I take this journey in writing this book I thank god that you are with me to go threw it.

NOTES

NOTES

CHAPTER ELEVEN

To Childhood My Friend
Dierre aka Red

Let me start off telling you how red has inspired me he has lived on his on for eight years he is independent as anyone I know he does not let his disability get the best of him his pholosphy in life is to do what u can for yourself even though he is disabled in the worlds eyes in mine he is not because he is determine to do the best for his self that he can possibly can do we now both live in apartments as neighbors and to red thank you for your friendship I will always treasure it god bless.

NOTES

NOTES

CHAPTER TWELVE

A Final Thanks

A final thanks to all those who help me put this book together and in this journey of telling u of how god has bless me a special thanks to Tierre King for his encouragement in this endever A special thanks to Mellissa Pittman for sticking it out with me threw the ugly years and encourageing me to write this book another person I would like to thank is Jason Rieth u have shown me and encouraged me to do my best and u showed me threw the tuff times I can make it A final thought has bishop a break threw today ministries and udca United Disabled Christian association I wold like to say to all of those that are with a so called disability just because the world looks at u one way that doesn't mean that the lord looks at you the same I hope this book encourages everyone that read it and finally let me thank the most important person of all the lord and savior jesus christ

NOTES

NOTES